How to Blend Essential Oils

Dr Miriam Kinai

Copyright © 2012 Dr Miriam Kinai

http://thebestsellingebooks.blogspot.com/

All rights reserved. No part of this publication may be reproduced or transmitted in any form or by any means, electronic or mechanical, including photocopying, recording, or by any information storage and retrieval system, without written permission from the author, except for the inclusion of brief quotations in a review.

ISBN: 1478334819

ISBN-13: 978-1478334811

Contents

1. What is Blending Essential Oils? — Pg #1
2. Top Notes, Middle Notes, Base Notes — Pg #2
3. General Rules for Blending Essential Oils — Pg #4
4. Practical Example 1 of Blending Essential Oils — Pg #6
5. Practical Example 2 of Blending Essential Oils — Pg #8
6. Practical Example 3 of Blending Essential Oils — Pg #10
7. Practical Example 4 of Blending Essential Oils — Pg #12
8. Practical Example 5 of Blending Essential Oils — Pg #14
9. Practical Example 6 of Blending Essential Oils — Pg #16
10. Practical Example 7 of Blending Essential Oils — Pg #18
11. How to Dilute Blended Essential Oils with Carrier Oils — Pg #20

1
What is Blending Essential Oils?

Blending essential oils is the art of mixing different essential oils so that you can create a healing mixture that has a pleasing aroma to your olfactory organs or sense of smell.

To make well balanced essential oil blends, you have to consider the volatility of the different essential oils and mix the essential oils appropriately. To do this, you have to know whether an essential oil is a top note, a **middle note** or a base note.

*****

2
Top Notes, Middle Notes, Base Notes

Top Notes

These are the essential oils with scents that evaporate the fastest and therefore they are first ones you smell. These scents are generally light, flowery, fruity and uplifting.

Examples of top notes include bergamot essential oil, clary sage essential oil, eucalyptus essential oil, lemon essential oil, orange essential oil, petitgrain essential oil and tea tree essential oil.

***

Middle Notes

These scents do not evaporate as fast as the top notes. They are generally spicy, herbal and balancing.

Examples of middle notes include roman chamomile essential oil, cypress essential oil, geranium essential oil, juniper berry essential oil, lavender essential oil, sweet marjoram essential oil, peppermint essential oil, rosemary essential oil and rosewood essential oil.

***

Base Notes

These scents are the slowest to evaporate and therefore the last ones you smell. They are generally heavy and woodsy.

Examples of base notes include rose essential oil, sandalwood essential oil and ylang ylang essential oil.

*****

3

General Rules for Blending Essential Oils

1. Decide what condition you want your essential oil blend or essential oil recipe to manage.

2. Choose approximately 3 pure, organic essential oils that can manage that condition.

3. Divide those essential oils into top notes, middle notes and base notes.

4. Blend your essential oils by adding 1 drop of the base note for every 2 drops of the middle note and 3 drops of the top note into a dark bottle.

5. Begin by adding the base notes and after adding each essential oil into the bottle, swirl it around and smell it before you add the next essential oil.

How to Blend Essential Oils

6. After getting a scent that pleases you, add the essential oils blend to the correct amount of carrier oil to create a healing massage oil or use them in your homemade lotions, handmade soap and hand poured scented candles.

7. These are not fixed aromatherapy rules and you can bend them to create your perfect essential oil blend. For example, you can blend by adding just one drop of each essential oil until you get your desired scent.

8. Always have a notebook at hand to record the number of drops of each essential oil you have added to create that particular blend.

*****

4

Practical Example 1 of Blending Essential Oils

1. Decide what condition you want your essential oil blend to manage.

Stress

2. Choose approximately three essential oils that can manage that condition.

Lavender essential oil, clary sage essential oil and ylang ylang essential oil

3. Divide those essential oils into top notes, middle notes and base notes.

Top note: clary sage, Middle note: lavender, Base note: ylang ylang

4. Blend your essential oils by adding 1 drop of the base note for every 2 drops of the middle note and 3 drops of the top note into a dark bottle.

5. Begin by adding the base notes and after adding each essential oil into the bottle, swirl it around and smell it before you add the next essential oil.

How to Blend Essential Oils

a) Put 1 drop of ylang ylang essential oil in a dark bottle, swirl and sniff

b) Add 2 drops of lavender essential oil, swirl and sniff

c) Add 3 drops of clary sage essential oil, swirl and sniff

6. After getting a scent that pleases you, you can now add the essential oils blend the the correct amount of carrier oil.

If the scent of this essential oil blend pleases you, you can add your blend to 10 ml of a carrier oil such as sweet almond oil to create a relaxing massage oil.

*****

5
Practical Example 2 of Blending Essential Oils

1. Decide what condition you want your essential oil blend to manage.

Depression

2. Choose approximately three essential oils that can manage that condition.

Rosemary essential oil, bergamot essential oil and ylang ylang essential oil

3. Divide those essential oils into top notes, middle notes and base notes.

Top note: bergamot, Middle note: rosemary, Base note: ylang ylang

4. Blend your essential oils by adding 1 drop of the base note for every 2 drops of the middle note and 3 drops of the top note into a dark bottle.

5. Begin by adding the base notes and after adding each essential oil into the bottle, swirl it around and smell it before you add the next essential oil.

How to Blend Essential Oils

a) Put 1 drop of ylang ylang essential oil in a dark bottle, swirl and sniff

b) Add 2 drops of rosemary essential oil, swirl and sniff

c) Add 3 drops of bergamot essential oil, swirl and sniff

6. After getting a scent that pleases you, you can now add the essential oils blend the the correct amount of carrier oil.

If the scent of this essential oil blend pleases you, you can add your blend to 10 ml of a carrier oil such as sweet almond oil to create a cheery, invigorating massage oil.

*****

6

Practical Example 3 of Blending Essential Oils

1. Decide what condition you want your essential oil blend to manage.

Arthritis

2. Choose approximately three essential oils that can manage that condition.

Eucalyptus essential oil, Lavender essential oil and Roman chamomile essential oil

3. Divide those essential oils into top notes, middle notes and base notes.

Top note: eucalyptus, Middle note: lavender, roman chamomile

4. Blend your essential oils by adding 1 drop of the base note for every 2 drops of the middle note and 3 drops of the top note into a dark bottle.

5. Begin by adding the base notes and after adding each essential oil into the bottle, swirl it around and smell it before you add the next essential oil.

a) Put 2 drops of lavender essential oil and 2 drops of roman chamomile essential oil in a dark bottle, swirl and sniff

b) Add 3 drops of eucalyptus essential oil, swirl and sniff

6. After getting a scent that pleases you or the total number of drops you need for that recipe, you can now add the essential oils blend to the other ingredients such as carrier oils.

*****

7

Practical Example 4 of Blending Essential Oils

1. Decide what condition you want your essential oil blend to manage.

Eczema

2. Choose approximately three essential oils that can manage that condition.

Lavender essential oil, roman chamomile essential oil and geranium essential oil

3. Divide those essential oils into top notes, middle notes and base notes.

Middle notes: lavender, geranium, roman chamomile

4. Blend your essential oils by adding 1 drop of the base note for every 2 drops of the middle note and 3 drops of the top note into a dark bottle.

5. Begin by adding the base notes and after adding each essential oil into the bottle, swirl it around and smell it before you add the next essential oil.

a) Put 2 drops of geranium essential oil and 2 drops of lavender essential oil in a dark bottle, swirl and sniff

b) Add 2 drops of roman chamomile essential oil, swirl and sniff

6. After getting a scent that pleases you or the total number of drops you need for that recipe, you can now add the essential oils blend to the other ingredients e.g the carrier oils.

*****

8

Practical Example 5 of Blending Essential Oils

1. Decide what condition you want your essential oil blend to manage.

Menopause

2. Choose approximately three essential oils that can manage that condition.

Lavender essential oil, clary sage essential oil and geranium essential oil

3. Divide those essential oils into top notes, middle notes and base notes.

Top note: clary sage, Middle note: lavender, geranium

4. Blend your essential oils by adding 1 drop of the base note for every 2 drops of the middle note and 3 drops of the top note into a dark bottle.

5. Begin by adding the base notes and after adding each essential oil into the bottle, swirl it around and smell it before you add the next essential oil.

a) Put 2 drops of geranium essential oil and 2 drops of lavender essential oil in a dark bottle, swirl and sniff

b) Add 3 drops of clary sage essential oil, swirl and sniff

6. After getting a scent that pleases you or the total number of drops you need for that recipe, you can now add the essential oils blend to the other ingredients e.g the carrier oils.

*****

9
Practical Example 6 of Blending Essential Oils

1. Decide what condition you want your essential oil blend to manage.

Premenstrual tension

2. Choose approximately three essential oils that can manage that condition.

Lavender essential oil, clary sage essential oil and ylang ylang essential oil

3. Divide those essential oils into top notes, middle notes and base notes.

Top note: clary sage, Middle note: lavender, Base note: ylang ylang

4. Blend your essential oils by adding 1 drop of the base note for every 2 drops of the middle note and 3 drops of the top note into a dark bottle.

5. Begin by adding the base notes and after adding each essential oil into the bottle, swirl it around and smell it before you add the next essential oil.

a) Put 1 drop of ylang ylang and 2 drops of geranium essential oil in a dark bottle, swirl and sniff

b) Add 3 drops of clary sage essential oil, swirl and sniff

6. After getting a scent that pleases you or the total number of drops you need for that recipe, you can now add the essential oils blend to the other ingredients e.g the carrier oils.

*****

10
Practical Example 7 of Blending Essential Oils

1. Decide what condition you want your essential oil blend to manage.

Acne

2. Choose approximately three essential oils that can manage that condition.

Tea tree essential oil, Lavender essential oil and Ylang ylang essential oil

3. Divide those essential oils into top notes, middle notes and base notes.

Top note: tea tree, Middle note: lavender, Base note: ylang ylang

4. Blend your essential oils by adding 1 drop of the base note for every 2 drops of the middle note and 3 drops of the top note into a dark bottle.

5. Begin by adding the base notes and after adding each essential oil into the bottle, swirl it around and smell it before you add the next essential oil.

a) Put 1 drop of ylang ylang essential oil and 2 drops of lavender essential oil in a dark bottle, swirl and sniff

b) Add 3 drops of tea tree essential oil, swirl and sniff

6. After getting a scent that pleases you or the total number of drops you need for that recipe, you can now add the essential oils blend to the other ingredients e.g the carrier oils.

*****

11

How to Dilute Blended Essential Oils with Carrier Oils

Essential oils are concentrated substances which should generally not be applied on the body undiluted.

They therefore have to be first diluted in carrier oils such as sweet almond oil, olive oil, jojoba, evening primrose oil, sunflower oil, canola, avocado oil, and apricot kernel oil to mention just a few.

The following are the useful formulas and approximate measurements that you need to remember when diluting your blended essential oils with your chosen carrier oils:

1% concentration

1% concentration = 1 drop of essential oil in 5 ml (1 teaspoon) of carrier oil

This 1% concentration is generally used on the face, by children and the elderly.

Therefore, if your blended essential oils mixture contains a total of 6 drops of the different essential oils you have used to make the blend, to create a massage oil with a 1% concentration that can be used for the face or on children or by the elderly, add the 6 drops of the essential oil blend to 30 ml of your carrier oil.

***

2% concentration

2% concentration = 2 drops of essential oil in 5 ml (1 teaspoon) of carrier oil

Therefore, if your blended essential oils mixture contains a total of 6 drops of the different essential oils you have used to make the blend, to create a massage oil with a 2% concentration, add the 6 drops of the essential oil blend to 15 ml of your carrier oil.

***

3% concentration

3% concentration = 3 drops of essential oil in 5 ml (1 teaspoon) of carrier oil

This 3% concentration is generally used on the rest of the body.

Therefore, if your blended essential oils mixture contains a total of 6 drops of the different essential oils you have used to make the blend, to create a massage oil with a 3% concentration that can be used for a body massage or a foot massage, add the 6 drops of the essential oil blend to 10 ml of your carrier oil.

*****

About The Author

Dr. Miriam Kinai is a medical doctor and a certified aromatherapist.

You can visit her blog at
http://www.TheBestSellingEbooks.blogspot.com/

or follow her on twitter at http://twitter.com/AlmasiHealth

Email enquiries to drkinai@yahoo.com with BOOKS as your subject.

Books By Dr Miriam Kinai

Aromatherapy Essential Oils Guide

Aromatherapy Essential Oils Guide teaches you about the following 10 commonly used essential oils:

Chamomile (Roman) essential oil, Clary sage essential oil, Eucalyptus essential oil, Geranium essential oil, Lavender essential oil, Lemon essential oil, Peppermint essential oil, Rosemary essential oil, Tea tree essential oil, Ylang ylang essential oil

Topics covered in Aromatherapy Essential Oils Guide include:

1. The characteristics of these 10 essential oils

2. The therapeutic or health benefits of these 10 essential oils

3. The different ways you can use these 10 essential oils

4. The contraindications or when you should not use these 10 aromatherapy essential oils

*****

Aromatherapy Carrier Oils Guide

Aromatherapy Carrier Oils Guide teaches you how to dilute aromatherapy essential oils with carrier or base oils and explains the characteristics and uses of the following commonly used carrier oils:

Sweet almond oil, Sunflower oil, Olive oil, Jojoba, Evening primrose oil, Virgin Coconut oil, Fractionated Coconut oil, Apricot kernel oil, Avocado oil, Rose hip oil.

It also teaches you how to dilute essential oils with carrier oils.

*****

Natural Body Products Series

These books teach you how to make skincare products as well as the benefits of various vegetable oils, essential oils, butters, and herbs to help you choose the best ingredients. These books contain recipes for normal, sensitive, mature, and dry skin as well as for managing cellulite, eczema, psoriasis, menopause, PMS, painful periods, arthritis, stress, sadness, mental fatigue, and insomnia. Books in this series include:

1. How to Make Handmade Natural Bath Bombs

2. How to Make Handmade Natural Bath Melts

3. How to Make Handmade Natural Bath Salts

4. How to Make Handmade Natural Bath Teas

5. How to Make Handmade Natural Body Butters

6. How to Make Handmade Natural Body Lotions

7. How to Make Handmade Natural Body Scrubs

8. How to Make Handmade Natural Healing Balms

9. How to Make Handmade Natural Herb Infused Oils

10. How to Make Handmade Natural Soap

11. How to Make Natural Skincare Products - this book teaches you how to make bath bombs, bath melts, bath salts, bath teas, body butters, body lotions, body scrubs, healing balms, herbs, and soaps.

*****

How to Plan a Cheap, Chic Wedding

How to Plan a Chic, Cheap Wedding teaches you step by step wedding planning so that you can know how to plan a beautiful wedding even if you are on a tight budget.

Topics covered include:

1. The Pre-Wedding Activities

These are the activities you should be engaging in once you decide that you want to get married regardless of whether or not you are dating.

2. The Key Events of any Wedding Planning Timeline

Understanding the key factors in any wedding timeline will enable you to plan weddings with a full year's notice or with just a month's notice without missing any important detail.

3. The Chief Categories of Costs in any Wedding Plan

Our wedding planning checklist will help you understand the key cost categories of all weddings so that you can successfully plan weddings of all sizes from large social events to small intimate gatherings.

4. How to Fit a Wedding into any Budget

*****

How to Make Fascinators

How to Make Fascinators teaches you how to create your own cone base fascinators, side comb fascinators, and headband fascinators.

*****

Managing Stress with the Word of God

Managing Stress with the Word of God teaches you how to manage stress effectively by combining time tested Biblical principles with medical proven relaxation techniques.

Topics covered in this book include:

1. What is stress?

2. What is the body's response to stress?

3. Symptoms of Stress

4. Biblical Principles for Stress Management

5. Medical Relaxation Techniques

6. Other Stress Relief Activities

*****

Rules Of Relaxation

Rules of Relaxation teaches you 130 simple relaxation techniques as it covers the A to Z of stress management from Assert yourself, Breathe deeply, Cast your burdens, Drink herbal teas, Establish social support, Formulate realistic goals, Guard your heart, Have complementary hobbies, Identify personal stressors, Jaunt, Keep the Sabbath, Listen to music, Meditate on the Word, Nab a nap, Optimize stress, Pamper yourself, Quash sin, Reason rationally, Schedule news fasts, Trust God, Use cognitive restructuring, Veto worry, Work out, eXperiment with aromatherapy, Yield to God to Zap job stress.

*****

Sword Words

SWORD WORDS teaches you how to wage Christian spiritual warfare using the SWORD of the Spirit which is the WORD of God. (Ephesians 6:17)

It instructs you how to wield your SWORD WORDS together with the full armor of God. It demystifies the enemy's devices and explains the battle plan. It also tells you how to position yourself strategically and communicate effectively with your backup so that you can win your battles regardless of whether you are fighting for your marriage, children, or finances or fighting addictions, opposition, and fear.

*****

Resolving Conflicts just like Jesus Christ

Resolving Conflicts just like Jesus Christ uses Biblical examples from Jesus Christ to King Solomon to teach Conflict Resolution Strategies, Third Party Mediation Techniques, Conflict Reduction and Prevention so that you can increase the peace in your home, the productivity of your ministry, and the profitability of your business.

*****

Christian Anger Management

Christian Anger Management teaches Biblical anger management tips and self help strategies to help you manage anger instead of letting it manage you and destroy your testimony, life, family, and career.

*****

Managing Stress for Teens

Managing Stress for Teens teaches teenagers Biblical principles, medical techniques, and life skills to manage 80 common teenage stressors.

It teaches them how to resist using alcohol, cigarettes, drugs, and how to overcome addiction. It edifies them to resist sexual temptation, fornication, pornography, homosexuality, and lesbianism. It also helps them cope with sickness, and disability.

Managing Stress for Teens also teaches teenagers how to manage emotions such as anger, anxiety, confusion, fear, guilt, loneliness, love, lust, low self confidence, and shyness. It guides them on how to deal with negative peer pressure. It also trains them to cope with family problems like abuse.

Managing Stress for Teens suggests constructive activities for teens who don't have money. It helps also helps them understand parental issues like pressure from parents and schools them on the best way to deal with bullying.

Managing Stress for Teens also clarifies issues on God, Jesus, The Holy Spirit, feeling they lack faith, and living right. It coaches them on how to deal with fashion trends, crime, corruption, and cultural practices. It also helps them understand puberty, their body shape, self image, gender realization and the effects of negative thoughts and words as well as helping them answer the questions "Who am I?" and "Why am I here?"

*****

Dr Miriam Kinai

Dark Skin Dermatology Color Atlas

Dark Skin Dermatology Color Atlas is filled with clear explanations and color photos of skin, hair, and nail diseases affecting people with skin of color or Fitzpatrick skin types IV, V, and VI.

Topics covered include Acne Vulgaris, Alopecia Areata, Anal Warts, Angioedema, Aphthous Ulcers, Atopic Dermatitis, Blastomycosis, Blister Beetle Dermatitis or Nairobi Fly Dermatitis, Cellulitis, Chronic Ulcers, Confetti Hypopigmentation, Cutaneous T Cell Lymphoma, Cutaneous Tuberculosis, Dermatitis Artefacta, Erythema Nodosum, Exfoliative Erythroderma, Gianotti Crosti Syndrome, Hand Dermatitis , Hemangioma, Herpes Zoster, Ichthyosis, Ingrown Toenails, Irritant Contact Dermatitis, Kaposi Sarcoma, Keloids, Keratoderma Blenorrhagica, Klippel Trenaunay Weber Syndrome, Leishmaniasis, Leprosy, Leukonychia, Lichen Nitidus, Lichen Planus, Lichenoid Drug Eruption, Linear Epidermal Nevus, Linear IgA Dermatosis (LAD), Lipodermatosclerosis, Lymphangioma Circumscriptum, Miliaria, Molluscum Contagiosum, Neurofibromatosis, Nickel Dermatitis, Onychomadesis, Onychomycosis, Palmoplantar Eccrine Hidradenitis, Papular Pruritic Eruption (PPE), Paronychia, Pellagra, Pemphigus Foliaceous, Pemphigus Vulgaris, Piebaldism, Pityriasis Rosea, Pityriasis Rubra Pilaris, Plantar Hyperkeratosis, Plantar Warts, Poikiloderma, Postinflammatory Hyperpigmentation and Hypopigmentation, Post Topical Steroids Hypopigmentation, Psoriasis, Pyogenic Granuloma or Lobular Capillary Hemangioma, Scabies, Seborrheic Dermatitis, Steven Johnson Syndrome (SJS) and Toxic Epidermal Necrolysis (TEN), Sunburn, Systemic Sclerosis, Tinea Capitis, Tinea Pedis, Tinea Versicolor, Traction Alopecia, Urticaria, Vasculitis, Vitiligo, and Xanthelasma.

*****

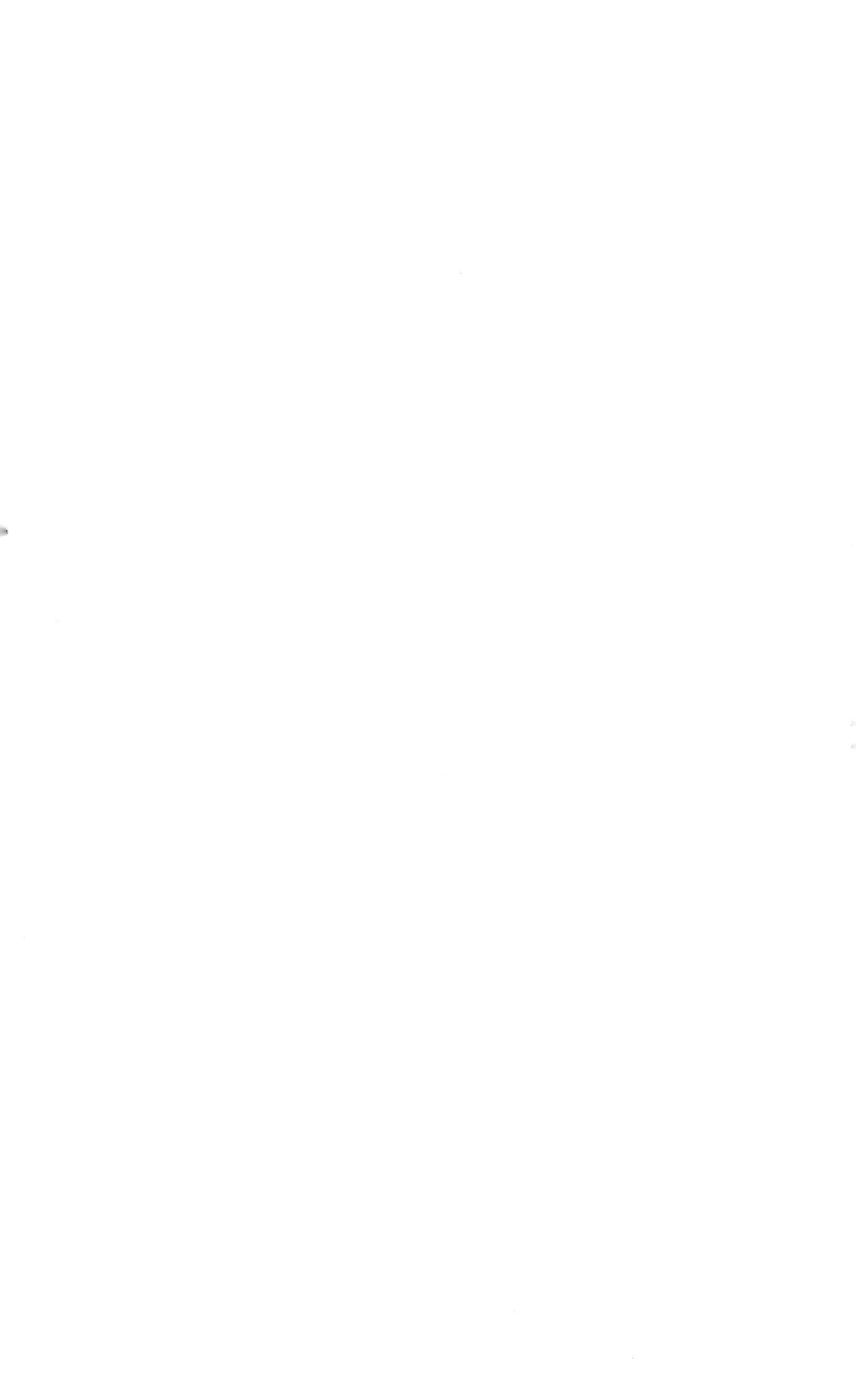

Made in the USA
Lexington, KY
31 January 2014